Make Exercise Easy:

Frequent Flashes of Inspiration

Lynn Kennedy Baxter, RN, MA

Dedicated

To you

The *Make Exercise Easy* series is not intended as a substitute for medical advice or care. See your physician or health care provider for recommendations about the state of your health, and your ability to exercise before starting an exercise program.

www.MakeExerciseEasy.com

www.BeConfidentToday.com

Contents

Introduction

∽∾

After smoking at least two packs every day for 24 years, I desperately wanted to quit, but my stress sabotaged every effort and I relapsed again and again. Like so many, I had repeatedly failed to kick my addiction.

As a nurse and psychotherapist, I understood the connection between smoking and stress. I had always been active and knew that exercise could help reduce anxiety, but exercise and sports were completely foreign to me. However, an unwilling mind and reluctant body were familiar territory.

I needed help to maintain my exercise program at home, so I created the *Instant Exercise Inspirations™ MP3* music program, which got me started and kept me going. Since then I have never had a problem exercising, in spite of illnesses, injuries, and the demands of a busy life. I also quit smoking in 1985, and have not picked up a cigarette since Christmas Day some 30 years ago.

Many years later, I became skilled in the amazing Emotional Freedom Technique, (EFT, also called tapping), which releases emotional stress, psychological blocks and barriers to create a better life. This simple and elegant technique effectively complements this system to incorporate regular activity in a positive lifestyle change. EFT dissolves the excuses and procrastination to exercise. *The Instant Exercise Inspirations™ MP3* fill the void and creates the ongoing enthusiasm and desire to exercise.

Make exercise easy!

Get inspired to exercise, and you can create an amazing habit. Combine these two techniques, and used them as instructed in *Make Exercise Easy with EFT* to guarantee the results you want. You can have the same experience of freedom to be a powerful self-starter through this innovative system.

"If you don't control your mind, someone else will"
— John Allston

Warning!

You cannot afford to have your mindless body be in control of your activity level, since the inevitable results are obesity, atrophy, and apathy.

Make Exercise Easy with Emotional Freedom Technique takes the struggle out of getting inspired to exercise. It creates a natural, intrinsic desire for activity by training your mind and body to want to move. It slays all the "dragons" of your excuses.

The *Make Exercise Easy with EFT* system with *Instant Exercise Inspirations™MP3* is an original, elegant, and unique system, which helps you develop a revolutionary, personal trainer for your mind that creates the desire for exercise and activity.

First, identify your personal, powerful, passionate purpose for making this impressive lifestyle change. Fitness has to mean something important and significant to you.

Next, dissolve every one of your sabotaging excuses, your dragons, with Emotional Freedom Technique. Chapter Two in *Make Exercise Easy with EFT* shows you how to do this. Videos are available on the companion website to demonstrate the basic tapping procedure and show you how to use it to slay your dragons.

Use the *Instant Exercise Inspirations™ MP3,* when you exercise. The companion audio program reinforces many positive attributes of exercise and bonds them to your body and the exercise activity.

Take powerful command of your mind, and your body in a positive, beneficial, and practical manner. These proven psychological principles create a powerful desire to exercise. You can have emotional inspiration and physical enthusiasm to be active.

You need to have a purpose for routine exercise. A habit of any kind, even exercise, can be deadening, unless it serves a greater goal. Find the result you want in your life. Identify what will free you, and you will take a big step in learning to inspire yourself.

"Exercise gives me energy; I have plenty of energy to exercise." When you say this enthusiastic command, for example, you cement the attribute of energy to the exercise activity, as well as to the good feeling in your body. This gives you more enthusiasm to continue to exercise. Find out in Chapter 4 of *Make Exercise Easy with Emotional Freedom Technique* why this works so effectively.

Use the *Instant Exercise Inspirations™* MP3 every time you do routine activities such as:

✓ Walking outdoors or on a treadmill
✓ Jogging or running
✓ Using the elliptical walker
✓ Bicycling on a regular or stationary bike
✓ Using the stair climber

To get the free recording purchase the book:
**Make Exercise Easy with Emotional Freedom Technique
&**
Instant Exercise Inspirations™ MP3

Use the *Instant Exercise Inspirations™ MP3* music every time you exercise a minimum of five times a week for a minimum of six weeks for the best start-up results. After that, use it as a booster when you need it.

Exercise starts in your mind. This system gives you the mental and emotional tools to transform yourself from couch potato procrastinator to a healthy, certified-fantastic fitness fan. You become your own best coach.

...And It Works!

The system is founded on sound psychological principles to produce results... and you will enjoy using it!

End your struggle to exercise now, because you *do* have the energy, the inspiration, and enthusiasm to exercise. You now have the independent power to motivate yourself. You can enjoy the extraordinary results you create.

Be among the first to embrace this new concept, and discover the amazing results first hand. What a generous gift to give yourself!

The examples in *Make Exercise Easy with Emotional Freedom Technique* are of real people whose names and circumstances have been altered to protect their privacy.

Best wishes for becoming a Certified-Fantastic Fitness Fan,

Lynn Kennedy Baxter

www.MakeExerciseEasy.com
www.BeConfidentToday.com

For Your Inspiration and Motivation

୭୭

This book of short essays on inspiration, motivation, thoughts, and quotes accompanies the primary book, *Make Exercise Easy with Emotional Freedom Technique & Instant Exercise Inspirations* ™ *MP3*.

Make Exercise Easy with EFT asks this question: suppose the Fairy Godmother of Fitness came to you with this proposal, "If I pay you $4,000 each time you exercise, would you exercise for 30 minutes a day, five days a week for a year?"

Wow -- a cool million dollars for a year's worth of exercise, with two weeks off for vacation! "Of Course!" is your quick, eager response. Who wouldn't jump at such an offer?

Flash! When it is *important enough*, you will exercise without any hesitation and with a great deal of enthusiasm. What could be easier? "I'm getting rich every time I exercise!"

Slay your excuse dragons with Emotional Freedom Technique. Learn how to tap away your dragons, and replace them with the positive change that you choose in *Make Exercise Easy with EFT*. This book also introduces you to the *Instant Exercise Inspirations™ MP3* to use while you exercise. There are 18 enthusiastic commands, such as:

Exercise gives me energy;
I have plenty of energy to exercise.

Exercise gives me willpower.
I have plenty of willpower to exercise.

Exercise gives me determination.
I have plenty of determination to exercise.

These commands cement a three way bond:

- ✓ The attribute in your mind to the
- ✓ feelings in your body as you exercise
- ✓ to the exercise activity.

The result is desire and enthusiasm to exercise, because these gentle commands take away the uncomfortable feelings in your muscles, when you start to exercise, and replace it with motivation to exercise.

You can say the *Instant Exercise Inspirations*™ to yourself as you walk, or jog, bicycle, use the elliptical, or stair climber.

Make Exercise Easy with EFT guides you through all of the questions to answer, and decisions to make, to create the most workable plans for you to earn that million dollars.

These questions and decisions include:

- ✓ Why don't New Year's resolutions work?

- ✓ What result do you want to get from your exercise?

- ✓ What is your personal, powerful, passionate purpose for fitness?

- ✓ How do you do EFT?

- ✓ How can you slay your excuse dragons with EFT?

- ✓ How can you make fitness doable?

- ✓ How can you keep it interesting?

- ✓ What are the four Trojan horses of fitness?

✓ How can you prime your pump?

✓ What is the power in your belly?

✓ Know thyself.

✓ How to use the *Instant Exercise Inspiration*™ *MP* music.

✓ Make your own personal, million dollar plan.

Regular exercise and fitness activity that is fun and doable is priceless to you and your health. Everything in your life depends on your having a healthy body.

Have some fun with motivating yourself. "Pay" yourself $4,000.00 every time you exercise with the checks on the following page and download more copies from the website.

Read the essays in this book from start to finish or thumb through the book periodically, and read one that catches your eye.

Enjoy!

Make Exercise Easy   1001
778 Energy Drive
Luvit, State of Fitness 80863

Pay to the order of_____ $ 4,000.00
Four thousand and no/100_____dollars

Bank of Motivation
156 Plenty of Time Ave.
High Intentions, State of Fitness 80863

Memo: *Today's Exercise*   *Your Fairy God mother*

Make Exercise Easy   1002
778 Energy Drive
Luvit, State of Fitness 80863

Pay to the order of_____ $ 4,000.00
Four thousand and no/100_____dollars

Bank of Motivation
156 Plenty of Time Ave.
High Intentions, State of Fitness 80863

Memo: *Today's Exercise*   *Your Fairy God mother*

The Power of Five

ক্ষৈত্য

The next five minutes will pass. It will pass quickly. You can use it for fitness or you can lose that time forever. Why not use the Power of Five?

In just five minutes, you can go from being a couch potato to taking an invigorating walk.

In just five minutes, you can do a complete body stretch and loosen up those stressed, tight muscles.

In just five minutes, you can do 10 reps with weights for five sets of upper body muscles; deltoids, trapezius, pectoralis major, biceps and triceps.

In just five minutes, you can change your mood from sedentary to active.

In just five minutes, you can stop eating a junk food snack.

In just five minutes, you can move your body and burn some calories.

In just five minutes, you can make an improvement in your exercise program.

In just five minutes, you can alter your attitude about fitness from negative to neutral to positive.

In just five minutes, you can burn 20 calories.

In just five minutes, you can change your life and become physically fit.

In just five minutes, you can dance your way to a happy mood.

In just five minutes, you can do 280 jumping jacks.

In just five minutes, you can deep breathe and relax, instead of stressing.

In just five minutes, you can run up one flight of stairs several times.

In just five minutes, you can make a different and better choice about exercise.

In just five minutes, you can begin to create a faster metabolism.

In just five minutes, you can make up your mind to do something physical that you enjoy.

In just five minutes, you can resolve to put your exercise plan into action now.

What would happen to your body, if you exercised the **Power of Five** several times a day?

Take Charge Now

ఞ∽ఞ

"If you don't control your mind, someone else will"

John Allston, Author

"Stomach, you rule!" proclaimed the voice in the radio ad for fast food and beer. It got my attention. That voice didn't want me deciding what was good for me. That voice was seducing my mindless stomach to make my decisions for me.

The fast food companies behind the highly effective TV, radio, and print ads that bombard you could not care less about your health. They just want you to buy their high calorie, junk food.

"Stomach, you rule," said it so clearly and unmistakably. You are a mindless object to be manipulated and encouraged to mindlessly consume fast food.

Take charge of your life, your mind, and your body now with exercise. If you don't take charge, other people will control you to act in their best interests. They know exactly what to say, and do to control your behavior. Their goals are not in your best interests.

Take charge of your life, your mind, and your body now with exercise. You can win this battle so easily, when you decide that it is, after all, your life and your body, and you are going to be in control.

Take charge of your life, your mind, and your body now with exercise. Learn how your mind works. You are more than your cravings. You are smarter than the people, who appeal to your spoiled inner child.

Take charge of your life, your mind, and your body now with exercise. Take back your power to make decisions that are in your best interest. Exercise. Enjoy a sport. Go for a walk. It's that simple.

Take charge of your life, your mind, and your body now with exercise. You can decide what messages are in your best interest and listen to them, such as the messages in the *Instant Exercise Inspirations™ MP3*. Learn how to resist the seductive messages that undermine your health and fitness program.

Take charge with *Make Exercise Easy with EFT & Instant Exercise Inspirations™MP3*. It gives you power over your mind and body to slay your procrastination dragons and instill positive messages to strengthen your motivation with fast-paced music.

s

The free recording of
Instant Exercise Inspirations™ MP3
is available with the book:

Make Exercise Easy with Emotional Freedom Technique
&
Instant Exercise Inspirations™MP3

Be Your Own Best Coach

ೞംഛ

"My mother taught me very early to believe I could achieve any accomplishment I wanted to. The first was to walk without braces."

Wilma Rudolph, 1940-1994,
American Track Athlete

On September 7, 1960, Wilma Rudolph became the first American woman to win three gold medals in the Olympics that were being held in Rome. She won the 100-meter dash, the 200-meter dash, and ran the anchor on the 400-meter relay team.

She was a basketball star in high school, who set state records for scoring, and led her team to a Tennessee state championship, before she went on to become a track star.

Born the twentieth of 22 children in 1940 in segregated Tennessee, Wilma overcame a premature birth weight of 4.5 pounds, crippling polio, and many illnesses as a child to become one of the most celebrated female athletes of her time. Her celebrity caused gender barriers to be broken in previously all-male track and field events.

Wilma married her high school sweetheart and gave birth to four children. She coached high school and college athletics, went into broadcasting, became a sports commentator on national television, and co-hosted a network radio show. She died prematurely at age 54 of brain cancer.

Now, why do you say you can't exercise, and why can't you work out? Remember Wilma. What would she say to you, if she were your coach? Can you remember, and take her coaching instructions to heart?

Be your own best coach for a lifetime of physical fitness, and enjoyment of sports. You can learn how to use outside support to develop your best internal coach for creating life-long fitness. You don't have to become an accomplished, award-winning athlete like Wilma. You just need to stay active and fit to have a great quality of life.

Learn to recognize the problems, doubts, pitfalls, negativity, and excuses you have about your fitness program. Tap them away with Emotional Freedom Technique. Learn to handle them as a moment of choice, and an opportunity for your expansion and growth, to achieve the fitness level you desire. Then you can successfully be your own best coach.

Motivation Day after Day

ৎৡৡ৶

"People often say that motivation doesn't last. Well, neither does bathing -- that's why we recommend it daily."

Zig Ziglar, Motivational
Speaker and Writer

Your lifestyle is made up of the things you do frequently, like sleeping and eating. Put exercise and fitness into the same category of activities that you must do day after day.

Stop grumbling and griping about exercise. You don't complain about taking a shower. You just do it, so you can be clean. You have the power to pay attention to the positive ideas and thoughts that motivate you to exercise.

Day after day you must focus on the benefit you personally get from your healthy, strong body; such as energy, confidence, and the stamina to do the things you love.

Pay attention to the personal values that are reflected in your goals for fitness. It is the power of emotional impact that makes a difference with motivation.

A friend recently reported that her 93-year-old grandmother fell and broke her hip. Unfortunately, her grandmother had been sitting day after day for many years. Walking for only 30 minutes a day would have kept her strong enough to prevent her fall.

This friend swears that she will exercise, walk frequently to stay healthy, and strong as she ages. This is the kind of emotional goal that will keep her exercising, so she put up a picture of her grandmother as a reminder.

Ultimately you have the power of choice day after day to stay motivated. You can listen to the motivating voice of the *Instant Exercise Inspirations™MP3.* Or you can listen to the whispered voice of your excuse dragon that seduces you into sitting and watching TV.

The desire for exercise day after day equals a healthy lifestyle of activity.

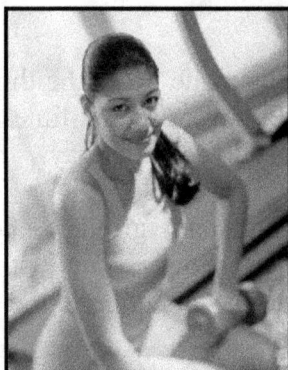

Just Imagine

ക⊱

*"It is time for us all to stand and cheer for the doer, the achiever –
the one who recognizes the challenges and does something about it."*

Vince Lombardi, 1913-1970, Football Coach

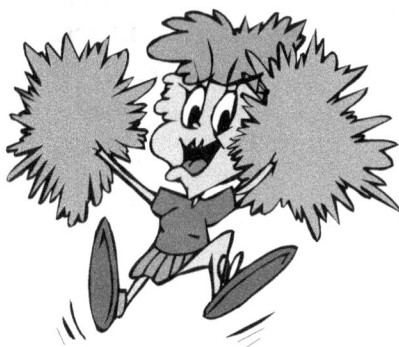

You are a doer. You are an achiever. You exercise, and work out. You recognize the challenges your fitness program presents and you do something about it. You don't whine and complain. You don't procrastinate too often.

You don't cop out.

You work out regularly. You exercise frequently. You incorporate activity into all phases of your life. You probably play at least one sport.

Stand up and cheer for yourself. You need encouragement to keep going week after week, and year after year. Fitness is a journey, not a destination.

Visualize your friends saying how tough you are as you climb 34 flights of stairs on the stair climber at the health club. They are so impressed with your stamina.

Imagine that you can hear strangers talking about how dedicated you are, as they admire your participation in sports.

Pretend the crowd is cheering you on when you play basketball, tennis, or golf. You get out there and do it, while others are making excuses.

Imagine your loved ones looking pleased, and being proud of you, because you exercise faithfully. They love you for taking care of yourself and for setting a good example for the rest of the family.

Just imagine you have a personal cheering section, your own pep club to help you create more energy to exercise. You have a wonderful imagination, so put it to work creating more of what you want – a healthy body and a great life.

Just imagine that Vince Lombardi really knew what he was talking about.

Footprints, Not Butt Prints

ల్లుల్లు

"You can't make footprints in the sands of time, if you're sitting on your butt. And who wants to make butt prints in the sands of time?"

Bob Moawad, Inspirational Author

Next time you think about letting your excuses keep you sitting on the couch, think about whether you want to make footprints, or butt prints. It is an interesting image.

You are going to make either footprints or butt prints. No way around it, unless you like to do handstands, or cartwheels. Then you can make handprints, which are just as good as footprints.

Get out there, and make some footprints today, whether in your shoes, or with your bare feet. Walk on the beach, jog, or dance to make those footprints in the sands of time.

Make footprints while you hit a few golf balls, softballs, or tennis balls. Throw the football around or kick the soccer ball.

Stomp around in the mud, and make some footprints in the summer garden. Rake leaves, and make footprints in the fall.

Make footprints in the snow as you shovel the walk, hike on snowshoes, or ski. The snow will melt in the spring, but your body will be in better shape.

Make butt prints, and the sands of time will grind you down.

Make any kind of footprint, and your body will know it, and the sands of time will be kind to you.

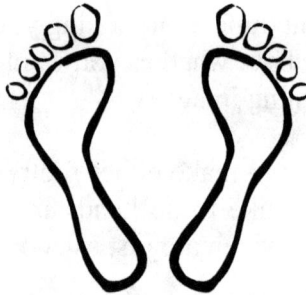

Go Straight

ဖာသ

*"The path of least resistance makes all rivers,
and some men, crooked."*

Napoleon Hill, 1883-1970,
American Speaker and Motivational Writer

… and fat!

Do you live by default or by goals? Do you take the path of least resistance, letting old habits or lack of thought define your way, aimlessly wandering along day after day in a mental, physical, and spiritual fog?

Your brain needs goals, because it is a goal-seeking organism. If you do not consciously, deliberately give your brain goals, advertising will create your goals for you by default.

Do you really think that Burger King or McDonald's cares whether you exercise or not? They certainly are crystal clear about their goals: to get you to consume the biggest hamburger, the most fries, and the biggest soda as often as possible.

Go straight. Set fitness goals that are excellent for you.

Go straight to Emotional Freedom Technique to overcome your obstacles to your fitness goals.

Go straight. Exercise with enthusiasm in the face of temptations to procrastinate.

Go straight. Say "no" to too many calories and too much fat.

Go straight. Determine what exercise works best for your body.

Go straight. Say "yes" to workouts that give you strong character and a strong body.

Go straight. Be determined to take the high road to fitness for your own sake.

Go straight to the *Instant Exercise Inspirations™ MP3* music and get the Inspirations you need.

The Power of Mental Muscles

ৎso৶

"Whatever you do, don't give up.
Because all you can do, once you've given up, is bitch."

Molly Ivins, Texas Political Columnist

Don't give up! You have the power to re-commit to your fitness program every day, or you have the power to bitch. Molly was probably referring to other things when she wrote this quote, but it is certainly true of exercise.

It is time for some strengthening exercises, and not just the physical kind. You need mental muscles!

Mental muscles are developed in several ways. First, remember your personal, powerful, passionate purpose, your compelling reason, and the million-dollar motivation that you identified in *Make Exercise Easy with EFT & Instant Exercise Inspirations™ MP.*

Make it easy to remember your compelling motive. Take a picture of yourself playing your favorite sport. Take a picture of yourself looking sexy. Take a picture of yourself with your grandchildren.

Put up a picture of a healthy heart. Take a picture of yourself lifting weights. Add the appropriate caption to your picture. Have some fun with this, and the payoff will be mega-motivation. Make several of these pictures for variety.

Put the pictures where you will see them: on your desktop, on the bathroom mirror, on the 'frig, on top of the TV.

Second, blast past the blocks and barriers that hold you back. Take back your power from your excuse dragons with Emotional Freedom Technique. Every time you give in to your excuse dragons, you give them the power to run your life.

Instant Exercise Inspirations™ MP3

Exercise gives me determination.
I am determined when I exercise.

Find the strategy to overcome every excuse that blocks you. Name your excuse dragon and get creative about what you have to do to slay it, and take back your power.

Third, talk to people who have incorporated fitness into their lifestyle for many years. They know that fitness creates something of great value for them. Ask them where and how they get their "mental muscles."

Fourth, use the *Instant Exercise Inspirations™ MP3* to get more mental muscles for yourself.

Be Bold

ço∽ego

"When you cannot make up your mind which of two evenly balanced courses of action you should take—
choose the bolder."

William Joseph Slim, 1891-1970,
British Field Marshal

Each day you are faced with many choices that determine the state of your health. Many of the choices are small, subtle, and seductively easy. "Take the stairs or ride the elevator?" "Burger King or Subway for lunch?"

Be bold in your decisions about your health and fitness. Take the easy way out in other areas of your life, if you must, but be bold about your fitness. Everything else in your life depends on your health.

Be bold for just five minutes.
Be bold. Don't allow yourself to make excuses.
Be bold. Take the stair and feel better about yourself.
Be bold. Don't procrastinate today.
Be bold. Walk at lunch.
Be bold. Make the energetic choice.
Be bold. Play your favorite sport on Saturday.
Be bold. Take the best course of action for your body.

Be bold. Say, "Yes" to strength training.
Be bold. Make your muscles and bones stronger.
Be bold. Turn off the TV, computer, or video games.
Be bold. Get moving. Just do something.
Be bold. Avoid having regrets about your health.
Be bold. Say "No" to veggin out on the couch.
Be bold. Burn 250 calories and then veg out.
Be Bold. Use EFT to slay your dragons.
Be bold in all the many small choices throughout your day. Let the small "be-bold-choices" accumulate in your health account.

One day you will discover that you are strong and healthy.

One day you will discover that you have become a bold person.

One day soon your body will reward you with excellent health and great fitness for your bold choices.

One day you will be a Certified-Fantastic Fitness Fan!

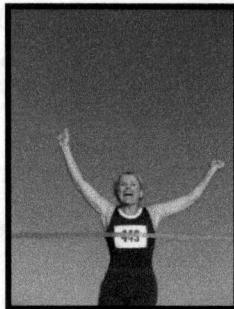

A Better Path

ఌఞఞ

"All one wants to do is to lie on the couch. From the couch - to the old folks' home – to the morgue. So, I shall begin simple stretching, exercise, and use EFT."

Personal communication from Connie, R.N.

You can join Connie and avoid the path from the couch to the old folks' home to the morgue. You are at that fork in the road ready to choose a better path. You want the vitality and aliveness you get from exercise.

Your path is healthier, because you practice a regular fitness program.

Your path is one of choice and responsibility for your health, not the default path to the morgue by way of fast food.

Your path is more fun, because you have the energy and stamina to participate in the activities you enjoy. Your path makes you strong, because you want the great quality of life that strength brings to you.

Every day that you exercise, you continue down a better path. You know how easy it is to go unconscious – to go from the couch -- to the old folks' home -- to the morgue. Just look around you at all the people on that path.

You know better. You put what you know into practice, so you are strong and healthy. You work out. You exercise. You engage in your favorite sports and activities.

You choose the better path with the help of Emotional Freedom Technique and the *Instant Exercise Inspirations™ MP3*.

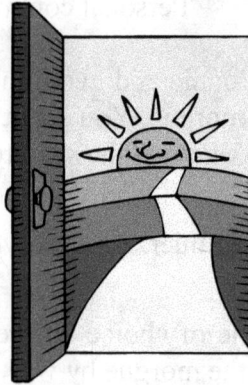

Why Wait?

৵৽৻

"It wasn't raining when Noah built the ark."

Howard Ruff, Financial Publisher

If Noah had waited until the catastrophe arrived, it would have been so much harder to build the ark. It would have taken too much time and would have been a horrible task in the rain. He might not have finished in time. A thousand things could have gone wrong that couldn't be fixed.

Why wait until you have a flood of weight or health problems to finally decide it's really time for you to exercise regularly? The smart person doesn't procrastinate too long before making fitness a habit.

All the research shows it is never too late to get the benefits of exercise, but the sooner you get committed to a fitness program, the less inertia you have to overcome.

Tom was a 60-year-old executive with a 50-pound Buddha belly, who just didn't think about exercise, until a heart attack scared the living daylights out of him. He survived, fortunately, but suddenly found himself having to build that ark from scratch.

No easy task at his age with all that extra weight. To his credit, he changed his attitude and changed his habits one day at a time. He became a new man and lost 50 pounds with diet and exercise, so his heart didn't have to work so hard

Make your "ark" able to weather the storms, and last a lifetime with plenty of exercise, sports, and fun activities. Get educated about the best ways to keep your ark in shape, remodel it, or maintain it. Building that ark gave Noah a lot of exercise!

The *Make Exercise Easy with EFT* is good for your "ark," so don't wait. Get busy today exercising with the *Instant Exercise Inspirations™ MP3* music.

Now you are in very good company, because you are not waiting until the catastrophe arrives.

Make Your Own Fanfare

ço∞છ

"No trumpets sound when the important decisions of our life are made. Destiny is made known silently."

Agnes de Mille -- 1905-1993,
Dancer, Choreographer

Special music signals extraordinary moments in the movies and TV. Enjoyment of the significant moment in the story is heightened through this entertaining device.

However, the dramatic interlude subtly leads you to expect and want the same drama in your own life.

It is easy to be disappointed by the lack of fanfare in real life. You make your decisions to be active in the quiet of your mind. It is important every time you exercise, but no trumpet heralds your workout.

No audience wildly applauds your determination to exercise for a healthy, strong body. Violins do not softly swell to a crescendo in the background, and play a triumphant finale at the end of a great workout, or challenging physical effort.

Now, through the wonders of modern technology, you can have all of that to increase your motivation to exercise. If you choose

31

to reach your destiny as a physically fit person, you can fulfill that destiny to the tune of the music you choose.

Use the *Instant Exercise Inspirations*™ *MP3*, say the inspirations, and then play the special music that keeps you doing your favorite fitness activity. Your preference of rock, country, classical, jazz, pop, or rap music adds zest and sets the mood for an energetic workout.

Find a piece of music with the horns playing a triumphant opening melody for the beginning of your workout. Better yet, find a piece of music like this, and play it <u>before</u> you start exercising, to get you pumped.

As you wind down, cool down, and stretch at the end of a workout, play music that signals a triumphant finale to your exercise effort. Play it in your head. Play it for real. Play some applause in appreciation for your good job.

After doing this for a while, the music you use regularly will stimulate the desire to exercise when you hear it. Important decisions may be made in the silence of your mind, but you can play the music out loud that makes you move.

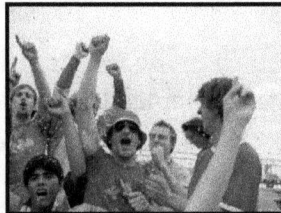

Summer Punch

ϣ∂ᐤᐤᘐ

Summer means hot weather for many people, which means that to avoid dehydration, you need to monitor your fluid intake when you exercise.

Try the following recipe for a Boost of Enthusiasm drink to help you and your exercise program:

- 1 two-liter bottle of fizzy "Just Do It" in pink lemonade flavor
- 1 bottle of concentrated Laughter
- 3 tablespoons of extract of Willpower
- Float exercise desire strawberries in the punch
- Serve over No Excuses crushed ice

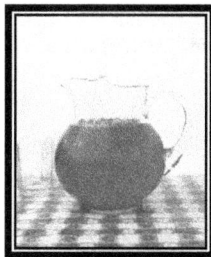

Here's another good recipe for Easy to Exercise sport drink.

- 2- liter bottle of "Yes, Yes, Yes, I Can" in your favorite flavor
- 1 liter bottle of Plenty of Time
- ½ cup of concentrated Desire
- 2 tablespoons of extract of Passionate Purpose
- Lace liberally with cherries of Determination
- Serve over No Excuses crushed ice

While you sip either of these delicious summer punches during your workout, favorite sporting activity, or household activity, use:

Instant Exercise Inspirations™ MP3

I have fun exercising.
Exercise is fun.

This will prevent dehydration and increase your enthusiasm for exercise simultaneously.

The Power of Potential

 formula

"Fall seven times, stand up eight."

Japanese proverb

How many times have you fallen off your exercise program? How many times have you let your excuse dragons win? It does not matter, because you have the potential to get up and exercise today.

Stand up, use your potential, and use Emotional Freedom Technique to slay your dragon. Work out, play a sport or go for a walk. Take charge of your health, exercise your power, and get the action your body, mind, and spirit need.

Exercise your potential to keep your body healthy and strong. Don't squander today's opportunity for exercise. The time will never come again, and you will regret the exercise you missed, because it just takes more effort to make it up.

Remember your personal, powerful, passionate purpose to go forward, and turn every excuse into enthusiasm.

All you have to do is stand up one more time. Give your power and energy to your exercise potential, not your excuse dragon. Refuse to be discouraged. That success energizes you. It enhances your self-esteem and self-confidence in all areas of your life.

Stand up and use your potential to overcome the seductive comfort of the easy chair. The easy chair may call your name, but it will ultimately leave you weak, feeble, tired, and living a pathetic life. It takes good health, strength and a strong spirit to live a great life.

Stand up one more time with the *Instant Exercise Inspirations™ MP3* and you will stay standing this time.

The free download of
Instant Exercise Inspirations™ MP3
is available with the book:

Make Exercise Easy with Emotional Freedom Technique
&
Instant Exercise Inspirations™ MP3

Pick Your Battle

ೂ∞ೲ

"Pick battles big enough to matter, small enough to win."

Jonathan Kozol, Educator, Author,
Advocate for Social Change

Fitness does not have to be a battle, but it is for a lot of people. You battle the dragons of not enough time, busy schedules, work demands, family demands, stress, laziness, and the couch.

If exercise and fitness are a battle for you, pick your battle. Don't pick one too big to win, too overwhelming to manage.

Don't set yourself up for failure by deciding you are now going to exercise for the rest of your life.

Don't declare that you are going to exercise for an hour five days a week, when you don't have an hour five days a week. That is a surefire prescription for defeat.

Pick a battle small enough to win. Pick a battle the right size for you. One size does not fit all. We are much too diverse for one size to work.

Maybe the right size battle is to start to exercise 10 minutes, six days a week, because that is doable with your schedule.

Maybe the right size battle is to walk for 20 minutes three days a week, because you can manage that much commitment.

Maybe the right size battle is to exercise 10 minutes in the morning and 10 minutes in the evening.

Maybe the right size battle is to get up 10 minutes earlier in the morning and win the battle over procrastination.

Maybe the right size battle is to banish boredom by spicing up your fitness with something exciting, appealing, and different for you.

What is the right size battle for you?

Use Emotional Freedom Technique to slay your dragons and win your personal battles, then use the *Instant Exercise Inspirations*™ *MP3* to keep you pump. After you win a few battles, you will be ready for bigger ones.

Be a Winner Today

ৎৡ৵৶

"You may have to fight a battle more than once to win it."

Margaret Thatcher,
Prime Minister of Great Britain, 1979 -1990

Be a winner today. Fight the battle against your excuse dragons. Understand that you may have to fight that battle over and over again, until you finally "get it." Fight the battle, and win it with Emotional Freedom Technique.

Be a winner today. Exercise, even though you say you don't have time. Eliminate that excuse dragon with EFT. You do have time for everything that you decide is important enough.

Yes, there are days when other things take priority over fitness. Yes, there are at least three days a week, when you can find 30 minutes for aerobic exercise.

Be a winner today. Fight the battle against laziness. There is a time to relax and recuperate, but just don't relax and recuperate all the time. Get up and get started with some activity. Stretch. Do a warm-up exercise.

Be a winner today. Fight the battle against "all or nothing" thinking about fitness. Add a little more activity into your life by taking the stairs, walking a little farther and a little faster.

Be a winner today. Fight the battle of being too serious. Make your fitness fun and enjoyable for you.

Add a favorite sport to your life or find one, even if you think you are not athletic. Add happy, snappy music to your activity. Begin to think of fitness in terms of play.

Be a winner today. Fight the battle with enthusiasm. Give thanks for being alive to fight the battle. Fight the battle so you stay alive, and have a great quality of life.

Be a winner today. Fight the battle with *Instant Exercise Inspirations*™ *MP*.

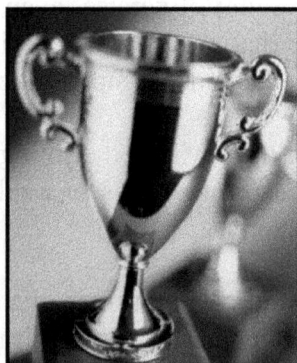

Split-Second

ക്ക

"Every great mistake has a halfway moment, a split second when it can be recalled and perhaps remedied.

Pearl S. Buck, 1892 – 1973, Author

Recall your decision to skip exercise today. You have a split-second, when you can still go forward with your fitness program. Seize the moment. Take charge of yourself. Exercise.

Don't make the mistake of letting your jam-packed schedule push exercise out of your life today. Actively decide when you will exercise. Make an appointment with good health. Make an appointment with your future.

Remedy the mistake of believing you are too tired. Go for a five minute walk first. Then if you are really too tired, stop; but if you are feeling better, keep walking.

When you lift the remote control to turn on the TV, which is not considered a strengthening exercise, you have a split-second to remedy that mistake. Drop the remote control, lift your body off the couch, and go have some fun. Go dancing, do yoga, try some tae bo or Zumba.

The folks who develop diabetes from being overweight, have a stroke, or break a hip due to osteoporosis, will look back and realize they made a great many mistakes.

They passed up a lot of "split –seconds," when they could have exercised to avoid so much pain and grief.

Grab that split-second in which your decision hangs in the balance. Seize the moment to change your mind. Now is the time to exercise before the day gets away from you.

You have a split-second to turn on *Instant Exercise Inspirations™ MP3*, a remedy for your unwise choice.

Yes, but….

ை

Do you ever catch yourself saying, "Yes, but…" when you know you need to exercise?

- ✓ Yes, but I don't really need to. I am strong and healthy.
- ✓ Yes, but I have work to do.
- ✓ Yes, but I don't have time.
- ✓ Yes, but I'm too tired.
- ✓ Yes, but not now.

You can "yes, but…" yourself into forgetting what is most important. Yes, you have important work to do. Yes, time is a problem. Yes, you are tired.

Yes, but - you are forgetting what is most important. Tell your Fairy Godmother of Fitness, "Yes, but…" She will answer, "Yes, but everything you love in your life depends on your body. You need your body to hug your kids, play in the sunshine, dance, make love, and even work long hours."

Yes, but – your passion in life depends on having a functioning body. Your body will support your passion for love, fun and work when you take care of it with enough exercise.

Yes, but – your personal freedom depends on your good health. Look around at the unfortunate folks who forgot to take care of their bodies. They can't go out dancing, or play golf, or climb mountains. Look at your own life. What you would miss if you were not healthy?

You can "yes, but…" yourself out of exercising, if you aren't careful. It is too easy to lose sight of the fact that exercise is essential. You can forget your personal, powerful, passionate purpose to exercise.

You can also "yes, but…" yourself <u>into</u> exercising, when you remember what is truly important to you. Exercise comes first, because you want a great life.

"Yes, but…" I need to tap away my excuse dragons.

"Yes, but…" I need to use the *Instant Exercise Inspirations*™ *MP3.*

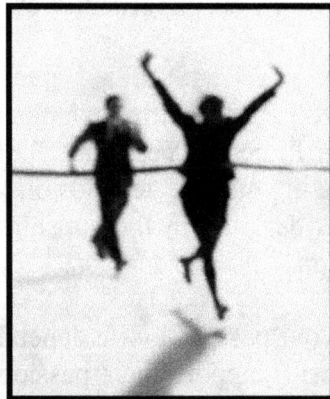

The Power of "Because"

ৡৢ৵

The word "because" is a powerful word, because the human mind loves to have a reason for "why do it?"

Reasons are powerful motivators for human action. The most powerful ones are also very personal.

Try these simple exercises to learn how to powerfully increase your own motivation to exercise, because you must have your personal, powerful, passionate purpose to maintain a fitness program year after year.

Picture yourself participating in your favorite fitness activity. Complete these sentences without using the word "should": "I played golf today, because…", or "I went for a walk today, because…", or "I rode a bike today, because…" What did you learn about your desire?

Do you tell yourself you <u>should</u> workout, play tennis, go for a walk, or ride a bike? Then complete these sentences. "I should play golf today, because….". "I should go for a walk today, because…." "I should work out today, because…."

The word "should" seldom reveals a truly personal, powerful, passionate purpose for exercise. There is another, quieter voice that says, "I should go for a walk today, because it's good for me, but I don't have time." In the fitness arena "should" is usually followed by "but," which drives away any enthusiasm.

Discard the "should" and stay with the desire, "I exercise today because…" This eliminates the "but," so you have your most compelling desire to exercise. Now you have the most powerful reason.

Over time, your personal, powerful, passionate purpose for exercise may change due to changing goals, events, desires, or age.

Sue had already taken up mountain biking, because she found it exciting. Then she blew her ACL (knee) ligament in a ski accident. Bicycling became an important activity in her rehab program, because she wanted her leg to be strong again. Her "because" changed to strength, so she could have the excitement of biking and skiing again.

Once you have your compelling "because," turn it around.

✓ Because I want a sexy body, I lift weights for exercise.

✓ Because I want to shed my stress, I go for a walk.

✓ Because I am going to live to a ripe old age and

✓ Because I want to be independent, I ride my bicycle as much as possible.

Because you know how to use this powerful word now, you have new power to exercise now. Enjoy!

Ghosts, Goblins and Spirits

૭∞∞

Which ghost haunts your fitness program? Is it the dark, faceless specter of "Not Enough Time"? Do the dismal failures from "Exercise Programs Past" return to haunt your exercise efforts now?

Which little goblin tricks you into abandoning your workouts? Is it the goblin called "Too Busy," that frightens away your determination? Does the troll named "Not Important," eat away at your intentions to exercise?

Does that ugly, twisted, little vampire called "Procrastination," grab your body, and suck out your willpower, leaving you lifeless on the couch?

Call upon the Great Pumpkin of Exercise and Fitness to exorcise those ghosts and goblins.

Invoke the Spirit of Health and Wellness, who has the power to overcome those little devils, to inspire you with a love of fitness.

Trick the ghosts and goblins that would put a hex on your fitness program. Treat yourself to an infusion of extra willpower with *Instant Exercise Inspirations*™ *MP.*

Trick the ghosts and goblins. Treat yourself to a strong skeleton. Do weight-bearing activities, like tennis, or jumping jacks.

Trick the ghosts and goblins as you walk your kids through the neighborhood at Halloween. Treat yourself and jog in place, or do a little jig to burn a few extra calories.

Trick the ghosts and goblins. Treat yourself to the time you need for workouts. Banish the specter of time scarcity, and the ghosts from past failed resolutions.

Trick the ghosts and goblins again, while you treat yourself. Get your priorities straight about the importance of exercise.

Trick the ghosts and goblins one last time.

Laugh in their face, because you are

       bigger....

          ....and stronger

             ....and wiser than they are.

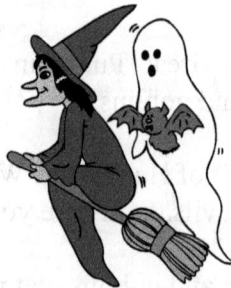

33.7 Million Times a Year

ೞ☙

You have an incredible muscle in your chest! If you are like most people, you totally take it for granted, even though you rely on it to sustain your life for your whole lifetime. You probably never give it a thought, until someone you know has a heart problem.

Here is what your remarkable heart does:

- ✓ Your heart beats about 65 beats per minute on average, and more if you exert yourself.

- ✓ Your heart beats at least 3,900 times an hour and at least 93,600 times a day.

- ✓ Your heart beats at least 2.8 million times a month.

- ✓ Your heart beats at least 33.7 million times a year.

Every decade your heart beats 337 million times, give or take a few hundred thousand beats.

By 70 years of age, your heart has beat approximately 2 ½ billion times; that is a "B" for billion.

If you live to 80 years of age, add another 337 million to that.

Your heart adapts to your needs. When you exert yourself, your heart immediately responds to pump more blood with oxygen, and nutrients to the muscles in your arms and legs.

When you slow down, your heart naturally adjusts and slows down, too. Your heart always takes care of you. Your heart always beats without any conscious help or instructions from you.

If you are wise, you take care of your heart and keep it strong with exercise.

The more you exercise, the stronger your heart becomes and the easier is for it to meet the normal demands of your body.

Athletes, who exercise a great deal, may have a resting heartbeat as low as 40 beats per minute. That lowers their heart rate by 38%!

How much wear and tear on your heart will you save, if you lower your heart rate by just 10%? You would save 3, 370,000 beats a year. That's a lot of living that you just banked for the future.

Use *Make Exercise Easy with EFT,* and the *Instant Exercise Inspirations™ MP3* to make your heart be strong, and shiny, and happy.

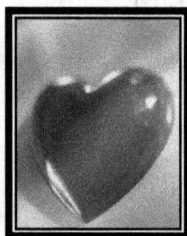

Keep It Up

ৎৄৣৣৣ

Hey, guys, keep it up! Your exercise and fitness workouts, that is. It's also good to know that researchers have found that regular, moderate exercise can prevent male sexual impotence. In this case, prevention is much better than treatment.

For 9 years, Dr. Irwin Goldstein from Boston University School of Medicine and his colleagues conducted a study that followed nearly 600 men, who initially had no problems with erectile dysfunction. They focused on lifestyle factors of smoking, heavy drinking, inactivity, and obesity that are believed to be the major contributors to impotence.

They found that men, who had been active to begin with, and those who took up exercise during the study, had a lower risk of developing erectile dysfunction.

Exercise appears to ward off impotence for the same reasons it can prevent heart attacks. Heart attacks and impotence both involve poor blood flow to the organ, while exercise helps keep blood vessels healthy.

In fact, ED can be an early warning sign of artery disease in the heart, since the penis is more sensitive to slow-downs in blood flow than the heart is.

Men who burned at least 200 calories a day through exercise were less likely than couch potatoes to become impotent.

That means that a 160-pound man needs to take two 17-minute walks per day at 4 mph or one walk for 34 minutes.

Speed it up a little bit to 4.5 mph, and 25 minutes of walking burns about 200 calories. Not that much of an investment to protect your sex life, happiness, and self-esteem, is it?

A word of caution: be careful about biking, since it may increase the risk of impotence. Bicycle seats can place excessive pressure on the prostate gland, and surrounding nerves, so check with your doctor, if you bicycle a lot for exercise.

P.S. A Viagra pill was consumed every 3 seconds in the United States, just two years after it became available by prescription in 1998.

Be careful, if you or your loved one uses Viagra. Seventy seven percent of Viagra purchased from 22 popular Internet sources were fake pills, which Pfizer, the maker of Viagra, discovered in a 2011 study. Most had half or less of the promised level of the active ingredient and many counterfeit pills were contaminated with toxic substances.

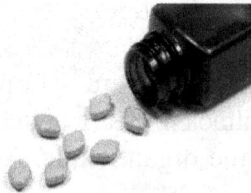

Reference: <u>Urology</u>, August 2000

Horrible Warning?

৩৽৵৵

"If . . . you can't be a good example,
then you'll just have to be a horrible warning."

Catherine Aird, Crime Novelist

This quote provokes a chuckle, but it highlights the choice you have to make every day.

Unfortunately, there are many people these days who serve as "horrible warnings" for too much inactivity and too much overeating.

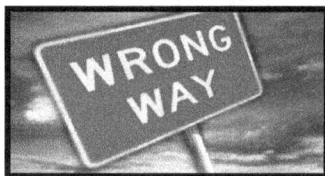

U.S. waistlines are expanding at an alarming rate. Data from the Centers for Disease Control show that in 1988, not one state in the United States reported an obesity rate over 15% of the population.

By 1998, 40 states had reached or topped that mark. In 2000, 22% of Americans were considered clinically obese. Today the CDC estimates 35% of adults and 17% of children are obese.

The researchers considered a Body Mass Index, or BMI, of 30 or greater to be obese. That means a person 5 feet, 3 inches tall and weighing more than 169 pounds or a person 5 feet 9 inches tall and weighing more than 203 is obese. The overweight folks at 25 to 29.9 BMI were not included in the above statistics.

Be a good example for yourself and your loved ones today. Exercise 22 minutes 7 days/week to reach that 150-minute goal. Exercise 12 minutes with weights in the morning before you leave the house, and take a 10- minute walk at lunch.

Be a good example for yourself and your loved ones today. Exercise 25 minutes 6 days a week to reach the 150-minute goal. Jump on a mini trampoline for 15 minutes in the morning, and take a 10-minute walk during an afternoon break, while you listen to *Instant Exercise Inspirations™ MP3* music.

Be a good example for yourself and your loved ones today. Exercise 30 minutes 5 days a week. Workout with a video for 15 minutes in the morning. Ride a bike for 15 minutes after work, while you listen to the *Instant Exercise Inspirations™MP3* music.

Be a good example, not a horrible warning.

References:
Centers for Disease Control and Prevention (C) in Atlanta, Georgia. The Journal of the American Medical Association, 1999; 282:1519-1522. The Journal of the American Medical Association, 1999; 282:1353-1358.

Muscle Math

૭ન્હ

Know your muscle math, because it explains the reason for weight gain, which is a result of both diet and aging.

The average person loses about one-half pound of muscle a year after age 35, and gains one-and-a-half pounds of fat. This loss of muscle can start much earlier, however, depending upon the person's activity level.

This change in muscle/fat ratio translates into 5 pounds of muscle lost and 15 pounds of fat gained every 10 years!

There is more to this story. Muscle is very active tissue, and burns eight times more calories than body fat, even at rest. Less muscle means a lower metabolic rate, so the rate of weight gain increases as the loss of muscle tissue accelerates.

When people diet to lose weight rapidly, they lose muscle mass first, which results in a slower metabolism. A slower metabolism results in rapid weight gain as soon as they go off the diet. This is the reason a dieter's weight will yo-yo. Dieting alone does not work in the long run.

Strength training is the only real solution to this problem. Stronger, bigger muscles result in an increased metabolism rate.

Aerobic exercise may burn calories and build cardiovascular

health, which is important, but the metabolic rate stays the same. Strength training protects you against muscle loss, when you cut calories, and protects you against muscle loss from a sedentary lifestyle.

Wayne Wescott, Ph.D., national strength training consultant, examined the effects of different exercises on the muscle/fat ratio in people at South Shore YMCA in Quincy, Massachusetts.

Seventy-two men and women were put on a sensible diet and divided in two exercise groups. One group did 30 minutes of aerobic exercise three times a week. The other group also exercised 30 minutes three times a week, but divided the time equally between strength training and aerobics.

Eight weeks later, the aerobic exercisers had lost three pounds of fat and a half-pound of muscle. The exercisers who also did strength training had lost ten pounds of fat and gained two pounds of muscle for a net loss of eight pounds. Very impressive!

Do your own muscle math. Be smart, and incorporate weights in your workout.

TV and Internet or Fitness?

ৼৡৼ

Do you say over and over that you don't have time to exercise? Or that it is really difficult to find the time for fitness? Think about these incredible facts.

✓ The average American watches more than 5 hours of TV each day and spends over 3 hours on social media.

✓ That is the equivalent of 76 full 24-hour days of TV per year, and 45 full 24-hour days on social media per year.

✓ By the time the average American is 65 years old, the average adult will have spent over 12 years watching TV.

✓ Between 1985 and 1999, 12 medical studies linked TV watching to childhood obesity.

✓ Fast food and food products are the number one television advertisements directed to children

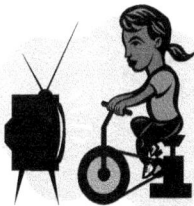

Take a look at your own TV viewing and see if you can find some time for fitness in-between you favorite programs. Get creative.

- ✓ Engage in some fitness activity while you watch!

- ✓ Lift weights, stretch, jump rope, do jumping jacks, floor exercises, and jump on a mini trampoline, or ride a stationary bike.

- ✓ Instead of heading for the refrigerator during the commercials, utilize that time for a little bit of exercise and stretching.

- ✓ Run in place. Run up and down stairs during the commercial or use the plastic steps from step aerobics.

Record your favorite programs, and eliminate the commercials to gain 15 to 20 minutes of time for each hour of TV. That's just enough time savings for a nice walk down the street.

Recording two programs per evening would give you about 40 minutes "extra" time in your day for exercise and fitness.

Check your Facebook and Twitter feeds, while you ride a stationary bike, or work the stair climber! You do have time to exercise.

Source: www.MarketingCharts.com
www.NYDailyNews.com

"Sex, Lies, and No Exercise"

ভেন্তর্ত

"Sex, lies, and no exercise" were the issues revealed in a study on men's health, to quote Alan Mozes of Reuter's Health News in June of 2000, reporting on the annual National Men's Health Week. In the year 2000 *Men's Health* magazine and CNN surveyed 2000 men on health practices and discovered these astonishing facts.

- ✓ 50% say they have no time for exercise, or are too tired, and over 40% say there is always something else to do that is more important.

- ✓ 50% said they would exercise, if they believed that it would result in their getting more sex.

- ✓ 30% are afraid of going broke.

- ✓ Only 10% are afraid of dying.

- ✓ 60% think they'll live to age 80, even though the average life expectancy for a man born in 1970 is only 67. Women still outlive men by approximately 6 years.

- ✓ 35% would not visit a doctor for chest pain.

- ✓ 25% would not go to a doctor for erectile dysfunction.

- ✓ 35% would be more likely to go to the doctor, if they were offered a free Swedish massage.

- ✓ 25% lie to their doctor when they go, because it is easier.

- ✓ Another 25% lie because they are afraid the doctor will get mad.

- ✓ Almost 35% lie because they are too embarrassed.

- ✓ 1 out of 5 will lie because they do not want bad news.

- ✓ 61% said they would go to the doctor, if the visit was free or if they could get in and out of the office in 10 minutes.

Many men only go to the doctor, if there's something terribly wrong. "We're saying to men that just the way you take your car in for an oil change, spend a few hours per week taking care of your health," said Ron Geraci, features editor at *Men's Health* magazine.

The message is this. Exercise and take care of your health so you are in condition to enjoy sex. We women love you guys, and want you around as long as possible.

Although this data is now 15 years old, I doubt it has changed very much.

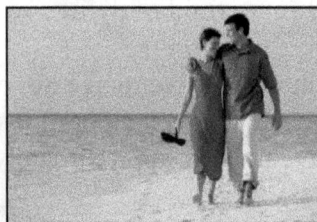

Heaven and Hell

ৡৣৡ

***"A lot of us try to get to heaven by backing away
from hell."***

Mariette Hartley, Actress

This certainly describes how a lot people approach fitness.

- ✓ Does fear motivate you?

- ✓ Do you focus on the health problems you might have, if you don't exercise?

- ✓ Are you afraid of heart attacks and broken hips?

- ✓ Do you beat yourself up for not exercising every time someone brings up the subject?

- ✓ Do you call yourself derogatory names, like lazy or slug?

- ✓ Do you constantly tell yourself that you don't have time for fitness?

- ✓ Do you frequently remind yourself, "It's such a drag to go the health club"?

Isn't this list of fears and negativity incredibly de-motivating? This is how people back away from hell.

Conventional Wisdom says: What you focus on expands. A busy mind creates what it is busy with. Focus on the negative, and you are in hell; this is not the path to heaven.

Stop, and back away from the hell of illness and disease. Turn around and face heaven.

Being in a healthy body is truly heaven. Exercise and activity will get you there. Change your focus to encourage yourself about any fitness activity that you engage in.

Start today. Notice what you do in the way of non-traditional fitness, such as walking from the car into the grocery store or lifting a small child, and add it to what you usually count as exercise.

Keep track of your progress as you become stronger, have more stamina, and feel better. Give yourself a "thumbs up" of congratulations or a pat on the back for what you are doing to get to heaven.

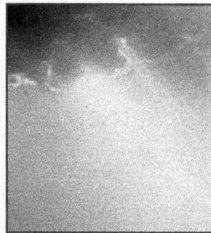

The Chains

ৡৣৡ

"Bad habits are like chains that are too light to feel, until they are too heavy to carry."

Warren Buffett, American Entrepreneur

The habit of not exercising, or not exercising enough, is one of those bad habits that is not too noticeable early in life. Youth has the distinct advantage of supple young muscles, strong young bones, and plenty of energy, if one has played outside a lot and not watched too much TV.

It is in the decades of the 30s and 40s that the habits of inactivity and physical apathy start to catch up with most people.

Low energy and a low desire for activity weaken bones and muscles. Bodies become fat and too heavy to drag around. Hearts become weak, and arteries become clogged with bad habits.

Pay attention now and notice the "chains" that are almost too light to feel. Do you want to wait until your body is too heavy or your mind is in a stupor to make the decision to exercise?

The complications of inactivity will catch up with you sooner or later. Those chains become shackles.

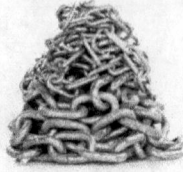

How much easier is it to increase your workout now, rather than waiting? Just a few years ago the experts recommended a minimum of 20 minutes of exercise, three times a week. Now the recommendation is 30 to 45 minutes of aerobic activity, five times a week. We know better now.

Fortunately, our bodies are not only responsive, but welcome exercise at any age.

✓ Muscles become stronger.

✓ High blood pressure drops.

✓ Stress hormones dissipate.

✓ Insulin-resistant diabetes is prevented or reversed, because cells need less insulin to use glucose.

✓ Bones are strengthened.

✓ Arteries are cleared of the "gunk" that can clog them.

✓ Hearts beat easier.

All this with a little exercise!

Break the chains of your bad habits now with *Make Exercise Easy with Emotional Freedom Technique & Instant Exercise Inspirations ™ MP3*. Get stronger and healthier with exercise, regardless of your past inactivity.

Don't Wait

ৎৡ৵৵

"I don't wait for moods.
You accomplish nothing if you do that.
Your mind must know that it has to get down to earth."

Pearl Buck, 1892 - 1973, Author

Do you wait for the "right mood" before you exercise? Do you procrastinate because you don't "feel" like exercising? Many people misunderstand motivation, and depend on the right mood to motivate them to take action.

If you do wait for the right mood, your exercise time will be spotty and your fitness program inconsistent. Often, it just doesn't happen at all. The body is tired or sluggish, so you are not motivated to go for a run, play tennis, or work in the yard.

If you wait until your body feels like exercising, you will be trapped into putting it off.

Don't wait for the mood. Get your mind in the groove of "just do it" when you say you are going to exercise.

Don't wait for the mood. Get your body going with action – any movement. Dance a little today for a change. Stand on your head if you are bored, and see what the world looks like from a new perspective.

Don't wait for the mood. Talk to yourself like a friend, or call a friend to talk some exercise sense into you.

You are the only one who can create the best mood, mental set, or attitude for exercise and sports.

✓ Do it through commitment and determination with EFT.

✓ Do it with the *Instant Exercise Inspirations*™ *MP3*.

✓ Do it by just starting to move - any movement.

Create your mood for exercise activity by remembering the joy of your body doing what you love – dancing, skiing, making love, tennis, and hiking, mountain climbing – you name it.

Do it by telling yourself to get going, and get out there with enthusiasm and music.

The Power to Persevere

ॐ

*"Our greatest glory is not in never falling,
but in rising every time we fall."*

Confucius, 551-479 B.C., Chinese Philosopher

Rise to fitness glory! Don't waste what you have started. You may have slipped in your resolution to exercise, but at least you made a start.

Keep going. Persevere. Rise up again, and again, if you fall off the activity wagon. Tap your way to rising again with EFT.

What can you learn from those times when you slipped that will help you persevere and rise to glory again?

✓ Did an excuse dragon jinx you?

✓ Did exercise go to the bottom of the list?

✓ Did you forget your personal, powerful, passionate purpose for exercising?

✓ Was it too inconvenient?

When you learn from the times you fall down, you can design a better, more effective activity program for yourself.

✓ What encourages you to conquer your excuse dragon?

✓ How can you make exercise a higher priority in your life?

✓ Have you identified your personal, powerful, passionate purpose for exercising?

✓ What have you done to make exercise as convenient as possible?

Use the times you fall off the wagon to leverage your rise to fitness glory. Experience the glory of your healthy, active body.

Stick to it. Keep up the effort. Progress, not perfection, is the goal. Make the necessary adjustments.

Get up. Rise to the occasion. Turn the situation around. All you have to do is exercise today. Surprise yourself, and everybody else.

Persist. Strive. Endure. Be determined to get up and do it again.

Use the *Instant Exercise Inspirations™ MP3*. Get immediate energy for exercise. The *Inspirations* bond the benefits of exercise to your thoughts, then bond your thoughts to the physical sensations you experience during exercise. It sets up a positive mind-body feedback loop that drives you to exercise with enthusiasm.

The Power to Live Longer

ᘒᕲᕲᕲ

"If exercise could be put into a pill, it would be the single most prescribed medication."

Dr. James H. Rimmer, National Center
on Physical Activity and Disability

There is a pill! All you have to do is swallow it. Now!

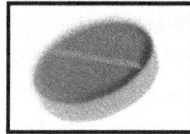

82% of heart attacks, and heart-related deaths in women, could be prevented, if they exercised, ate well, and didn't smoke, according to Dr. Meir J. Stampfer, and a team of researchers at Harvard Medical School in Boston, Massachusetts.

Dr. Stampfer's team studied 84,129 healthy female nurses for 14 years, examining the association between heart disease and lifestyle. They defined a low-risk lifestyle as:

✓ Moderate exercise at least 30 minutes a day.

✓ High-fiber diet that is low in saturated fats.

✓ Normal weight.

✓ Drink at least half an alcoholic drink a day, if not alcoholic.

✓ Do not smoke.

The bad news was that only 3% of the women in the study lived a healthy lifestyle.

The good news was that this healthy group was 80% less likely to have a heart attack, or die of heart disease, than the other 97%, even after factoring in age, cholesterol level, and family history of heart disease.

Heart disease remains the number one killer of both men and women in the United States. Researchers do not dispute that drugs to lower cholesterol and high blood pressure can prevent heart disease, but these drugs are expensive, and often have unwanted side effects.

"Adopting a healthier lifestyle could prevent a substantial majority of coronary disease events in women," the researchers concluded in an article in the prestigious *New England Journal of Medicine*, July 2000.

This lifestyle "pill" is inexpensive, even cheap, when measured against the cost of medication, a heart attack, disability or death.

Exercise moderately for 30 minutes a day. Your heart will thank you. Your loved ones will thank you. You will feel so good about yourself for having the foresight to implement this research in your own life.

….and you will live longer, too.

Get To Paradise

ϛ๑๛

"If you want to get to paradise, you have to pedal."

Chicken Run, The Movie

Great advice and a good laugh from a bird that cannot fly, for those of you who have not seen this movie for kids.

This quote is a truism from a chicken flying the coop in this children's Claymation version of *The Great Escape.*

Any place worth getting to is going to take some effort. Repeated, determined, frequent effort. The same is true of your fitness program. Work and effort are a necessary part of creating the physical fitness that supports your health and activities.

Effort is required to escape the flabby muscles, stiffness, and fatigue of being cooped up in front of a computer or the TV.

Effort, ingenuity and EFT tapping are necessary to find the way out of your own, personal prison of excuses that you use to avoid exercising.

The prison is in your head, just as Ginger, the persistent leader of the chicken escape, says. Believing you can do it, even if you have tried and failed before, is essential.

Figure out how you can best "pedal" your way to paradise. Walk, run, jog, cycle, row, lift, jump, and swing dance – it doesn't matter, as long as you make the effort 30 minutes a day, most days.

Every time you "pedal" or expend some effort in exercise, think about your paradise, the one that you are working toward.

Some people's paradise will be a body that is buff and sexy. Some people's paradise will be a body that is flexible and strong. Another's version of paradise will be a body with the energy and physical skill to enjoy their favorite sport. Still others are looking for the paradise of staying youthful.

You have to know what your version of paradise looks like. Otherwise, how will you know when you get there?

Remember the chickens from *Chicken Run,* who escaped the certain death of being cooked in potpies?

Escape your own "pot" as you pedal your way to paradise.

If I'd Known...

ی‌و‌رى

*"If I'd known I was going to live this long,
I would've taken better care of myself."*

Conventional Wisdom

In 1900, you could expect to live for approximately 49 years. Infectious diseases were the biggest cause of death, if you survived infancy. Many children didn't survive. In fact between 10% and 20% of children died before their first birthday.

Fast-forward more than a century. By 2010 you could expect to live to age 78. The infant mortality rate in the USA had dropped to 1%. Chronic illnesses like heart disease and cancer are the major causes of death.

We are living longer, 60% longer than 1900, because of better medicine, and drastically improved public health practices.

If you knew when you bought a new car that it was going to have to last you 400,000 miles, you would naturally take good care of it. You would drive it carefully, change the oil on schedule, and get it tuned up regularly. You would keep it in good working condition, because you are a smart person.

Your "manufacturer's manual" strongly suggests that you do your part to make your own "vehicle," last a long time. It is a great model and you are going to need it for 70 to 80, maybe 90 years, if you were blessed with a good model.

Exercise is absolutely essential for the proper working condition of this model. Exercise maintains a healthy heart muscle and good muscle tone, great blood pressure, normal blood sugar, strong bones, energy, stamina, and much more.

This model has a phenomenal self-repairing program built into it. Simply engage in moderate physical activity for 30 minutes a day to activate that program.

Consume only the number of calories necessary for basic metabolism and activity. Get enough rest. Enjoy life with friends, because this model thrives on happiness.

Even if you have neglected your vehicle, and it is in poor condition, you can make up for that now. Exercise enough to jump-start the self-repairing program, and kick it into high gear.

Do your part to be blessed with a long life, a healthy life, and a great quality of life with *Instant Exercise Inspirations™ MP3*.

Exercise on a regular basis, and do it now before it is too late, even if you think you are too young.

Now you know - you are going to live that long!

Please Tell Me

I love to hear your stories, your struggles and your successes in making these lifestyle changes for yourself.

Please write to me at:
Stories@MakeExerciseEasy.com

Helps other readers find a way to make these important lifestyle changes. Please post your brief review and a rating on Amazon and send me your comments. It only takes about a minute to help another person.

This is the companion book to:

Make Exercise Easy with Emotional Freedom Technique
& Instant Exercise Inspirations™ MP3

Visit my author page, Lynn Kennedy Baxter,

on Amazon.

Also available from Lynn Kennedy Baxter:

Make Exercise Easy: Tapping & Activity Journal

Supercharge Your Affirmations with EFT

www.ingramcontent.com/pod-product-compliance
Lightning Source LLC
Chambersburg PA
CBHW050555280326
41933CB00011B/1897

9 780692 412329